This book i

_____

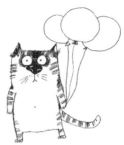

I think you're an amazing healthcare
worker and awesome human being.
You deserve all the recognition that
you can get.
Thank you.

From:

_____

£1 from the sale of this book, will be
donated to NHS Charities Together
(registered charity no. 1186569)

NHS CHARITIES
TOGETHER

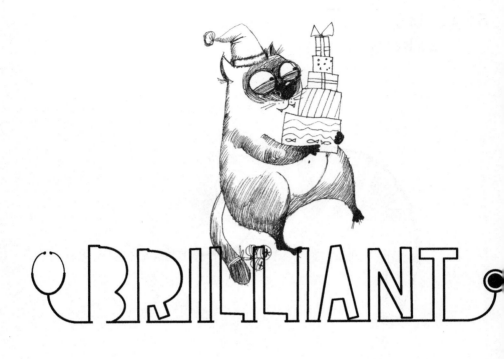

BRILLIANT

We all need a reminder of how brilliant we are now and again.

Today, you deserve a reminder more than most.

Some days are busy, and you might feel like you are spinning plates.

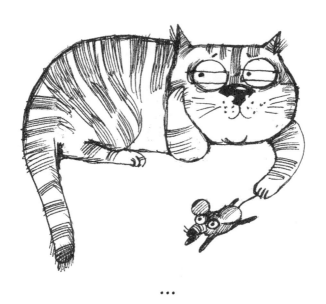

...

Or maybe you seem to have projects coming out of your ears...

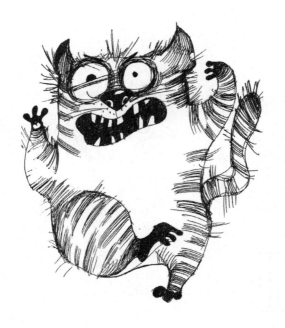

Sometimes that pesky critic appears on our shoulder to tell us about everything that we've 'missed' and where we should have done better.

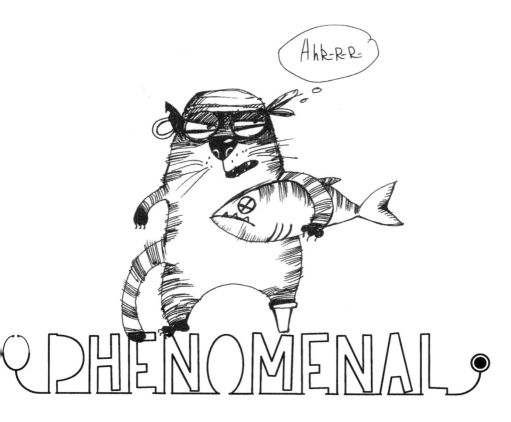

PHENOMENAL

..Or some days you might feel like a bit of an imposter when praised or progressing (you're not one).

So many people are grateful for the phenomenal work that you do every day, even the things that might seem like no big deal.

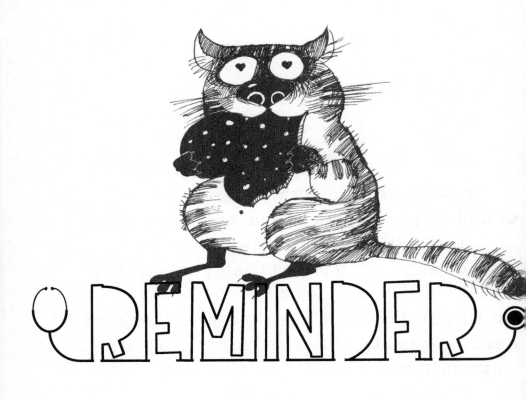

Here's your reminder that you ARE
valuable.
And amazing.
And brilliant.
And appreciated.
Someone wants to let you know that
today.

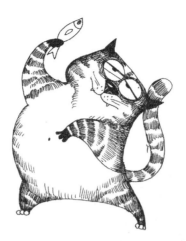

You're an awesome life-saving,
wound-dressing, illness treating hero.
In fact, you might even be an
ambulance driving, first responding
hero.
Or maybe you're a theatre and surgery
hero, a health visitor hero, a GP hero,
nurse hero, an admin or management
hero, or a cleaning hero.
You see, healthcare heroes come in many
guises.
From neurosurgery to ophthalmology,
from A&E to therapy.
Whatever your sector, you're changing
lives every day.
You have your own unique set of
experiences, that will never be the
same as anyone else's.

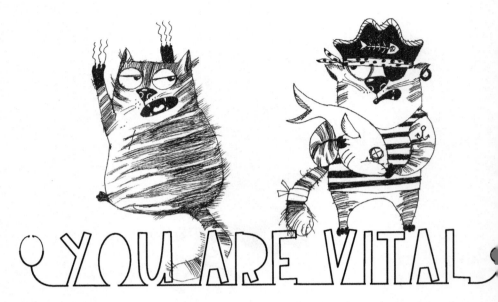

YOU ARE VITAL

Sometimes we forget about that uniquenes

We are often quick to see the parts tha
our job roles do not entail, and forget
that we are all vital.

Inside and outside of work, it is easy t
get drawn into the comparison trap.

Whether that's comparing on social medi
or seeing others from our graduate yea
doing amazing things (and forget that
maybe they feel envious of our
achievements).

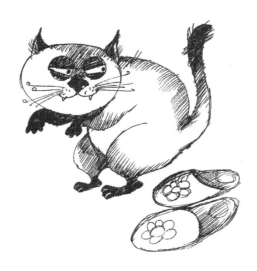

Eleanor Roosevelt said "comparison is
the thief of joy" and oh boy was she
right.
The odds of a human being born were
calculated at 1 in 400 trillion.
Wow.
You're the only you on Earth, you just
happen to be in healthcare too.
You're totally unique (and valuable).
How special is that?
You can't compare unique, so why bother
trying?

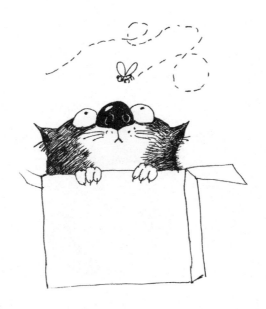

In this uniqueness are some amazing
strengths and qualities.
Sometimes we forget those too.
The person who sent you this book can
see them all too well.
Realign with your strengths, spend some
time to soak up your triumphs (of which
there are plenty).
There are thousands of lives that have
changed because of you.
Be kind to yourself.

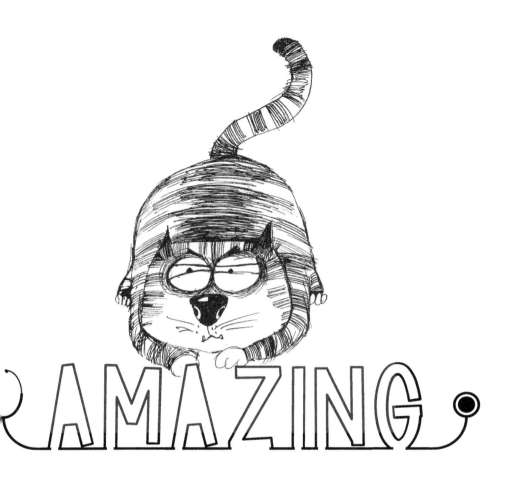

How can we be kind to ourselves?
Let's remember we don't have to
believe everything that we think.
Sometimes we all have that inner
critic that pipes up to doubt us.

You're doing a great job, and
amazing work.

www.katiefordvet.com

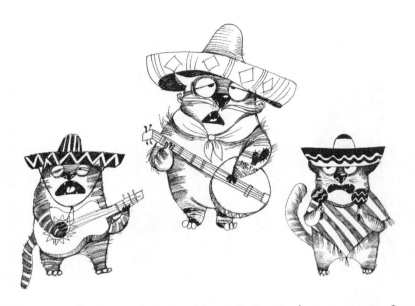

And how else can we be kind to ourselves?
Nourish yourself.
Set time aside for this amazing person to
recharge.
Find what works for you.
Mindfulness or meditation?
Maybe you're a yogi, or a runner.
Perhaps you're a crafter.
What if you're an adrenaline junkie?
Or a skier, or even part of a Mexican band?
Perhaps adding a weekly massage is a must.
For some that might include medications or
therapy.
You do you.
You totally deserve it.

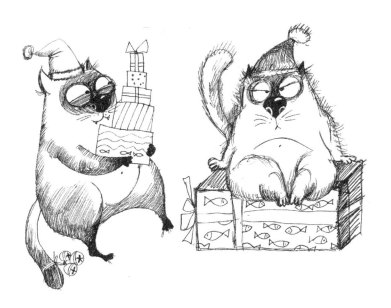

On the topic of being kind, let's be
kind to each other too.
Make the extra cuppa.
Check in with your colleagues.
Let's try to see other perspectives
too.
We never know what's going on for
anyone else.
You're all amazing members of the
team.
#bekind (always)

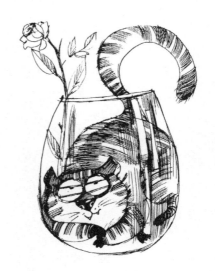

It's ok not to know something.... at any stage in your journey.

Let's remember we work in teams and are here to help each other build our knowledge.

We always know how much you care.

Equally, failing doesn't make you a failure.

At the times of failure, we often have our greatest lessons.

Ask: what can I learn from this?

What would your best friend say to you?

Let's start speaking to ourselves in that way too.

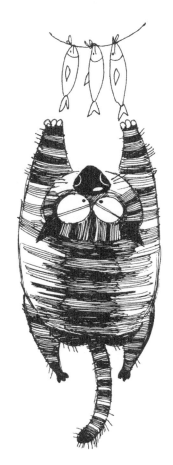

Sometimes being kind to ourselves is asking for help.
This might be for work, for home life, or when we don't feel ourselves.
You are all healthcare superheroes, but even Superman was Clark Kent for some of the day.
You don't have to know everything, nobody does.

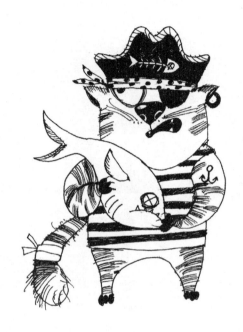

We are the captain of our ship, the maste
of our fate*.
(*but we don't have to sail alone)

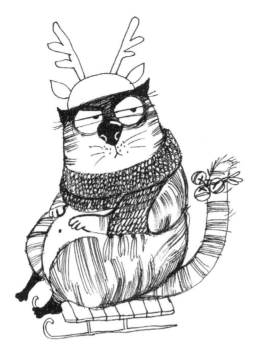

The email saying you secretly failed
your exams is NOT on its way.

You earned the praise and
qualifications, it was not by mistake.
You're changing lives every day,
whether you're prescribing medication
or ensuring wards are clean.

70% of the population have
experienced feeling like an imposter
.... we simply can't all be frauds.
Not even you*.
(*or you!)

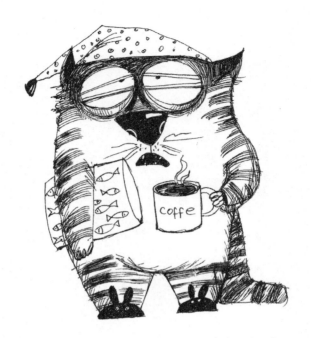

Some days will be tricky.
Some days you will be pulled in 87
different directions.
But keep your focus on what matters.
Find joy in the small things.
The smiles, the thanks, how far
you've come.
The cards and messages.
The laughs with your colleagues.
The differences that you make every
day, even when you forget.
Find time for gratitude.
Find time for you too.
Your work is appreciated.

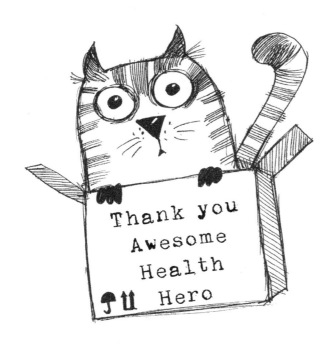

Thank you
Awesome
Health
Hero

Whilst we're on the topic of thanks.
Accept the compliments.
Try to stop the "yeah, but"s.
The thanks is justified, even as part of
a team, you can share with them too, but
soak up your contribution.
It's their thanks to give, they made that
decision, receive it graciously.

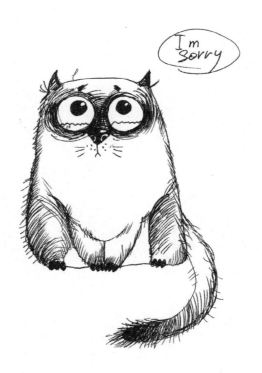

The ones who complain and say things
they'd later regret - let's not give our
power to them.
None of us ever know the full story.
Maybe they had a bad day too.
This doesn't excuse it, but might
explain it.
We're all human.
We're sorry for the things people said
that they probably don't mean.
Let's keep coming back to kindness.

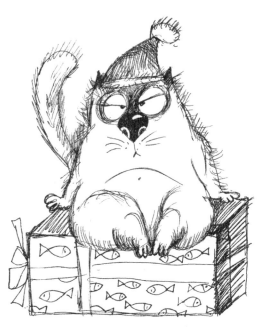

There are so many people out there
that are grateful for the differences
that you've made, not just the person
sending this book.
The lives you've saved.
The wounds you've healed.
The days you've brightened up.
The ones you've helped in difficult
circumstances.
The times you've been a reassuring
voice on the end of the phone.

Remember those ones, they definitely
remember you.

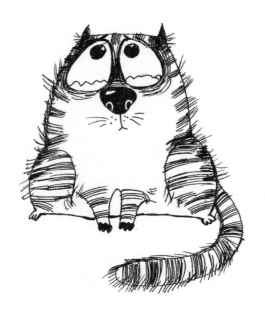

Ask yourself: what went well today?
Be your own cheerleader, look for the
good.
It might seem tricky at first, but
give it a try.
Give yourself some credit, you
deserve it.
Lots of people think that you do.

(And we'll be here cheering you in the
meantime.)

www.katiefordvet.com

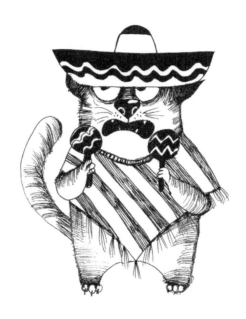

And whilst we are talking about credit....
Maybe there was once a time you doubted you'd ever do the job that you do.
You did it.
It takes a special person, and that person is you.

You're so full of potential to grow, but you're still valuable all the same.

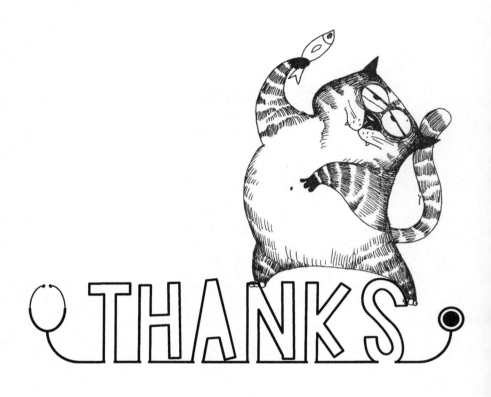

THANKS

You do so many amazing things every
day that you might take for granted.
You have impacted so many lives, young
and old.
You are a skilled healthcare wizard.
A&E or Paediatrics.
Therapy or Radiography.
Management or Midwifery.
Pathology or Support.
Student or retired.
This remains true.
Soak that up.

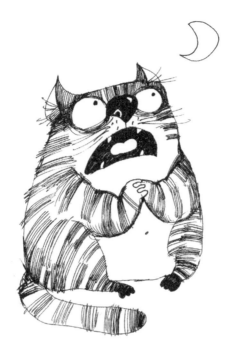

Sometimes the Sunday Scaries rear
their head.
"What if there's been a disaster over
the weekend?"
"What if I've made a mistake?"
"What if Monday throws me something
I can't handle?"
Change the 'what if' to 'even if'.
Even if something unexpected
happens, you'll work through it as a
team.

www.katiefordvet.com

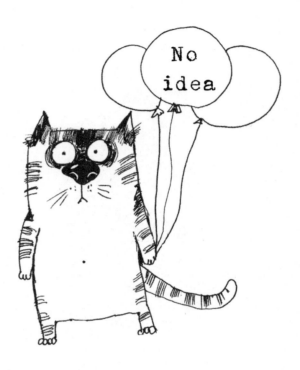

From time to time you won't have a clue
what to do.
That's ok.
Someone else will know... reach out.
Have faith in your skillset too.
Reflect back and give yourself some
credit when you overcome the obstacle,
even with help.
This is where we grow.

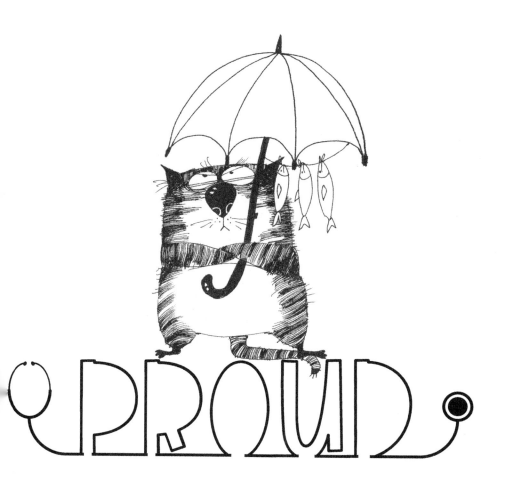

We've seen you working so hard, and that is only the tip of the healthcare iceberg.
We are proud.
And appreciative.
You are so valuable.

www.katiefordvet.com

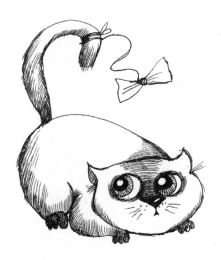

On that topic....you're valuable,
not because of the letters after your
name, however many there may be.
Or because of where you work.
Or because of the car that you drive,
or the extra certificates that you
have.
Plenty of people think you're
valuable...
....just because you're you*.

(*even on the days where you don't get out from under
the duvet and watch TV all day)

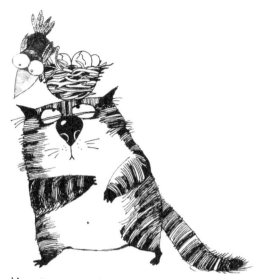

And don't forget that being you
involves so much more than your job
title.
You're a son or a daughter, and maybe
a sibling, a cousin, perhaps a mother
or a father, or partner.
There are many facets to you.
You'll have your own set of things
that make you happy.
Always remember to embrace those
things.
You're allowed happiness, and not on a
delayed payment plan.
Try to spend time on all of you, as
well as your career.

www.katiefordvet.com

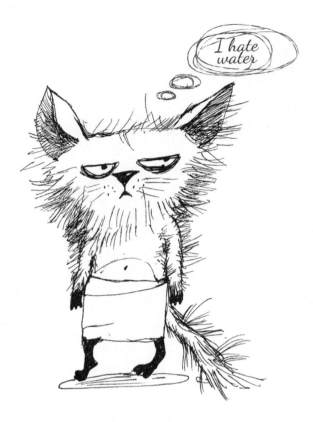

I hate water

Look after that amazing person.
Be kind to yourself.
You cannot pour from an empty
cup.
You're allowed to stop and have
a break when you need to.
In fact, we suggest you go and
pour yourself a brew.
Grab a biscuit too if you like.

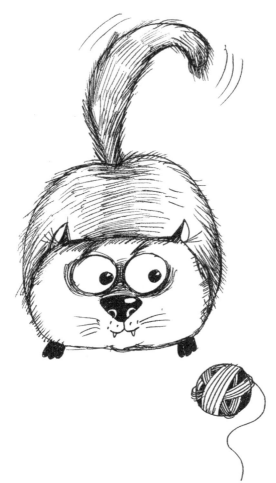

So this has been your reminder:
You are an amazing, unique, valuable
human being that has their own
individual journey, who just happens
to be an amazing healthcare hero too.
Remember that.

And one final time: thank you.

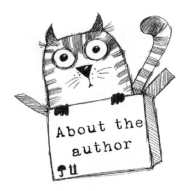

About the author

This little book was brought to you by Dr. Katie Ford, a veterinary surgeon, speaker and coach. Katie had her own journey with self-doubt and imposter syndrome as a vet, despite external success. Although not the same, parallels can be drawn between veterinary and medical industries, and "To an amazing healthcare worked" stemmed from a veterinary version of the book: we thought healthcare heroes deserved the same reminders.

Thank you for all of your incredible work.

You can read more about Katie at www.katiefordvet.com. @katiefordvet

Could you pass this on to someone else that needs this reminder next?

Images on commercial license from Tatiana Davidova at Creative Market.
Fonts: CLN Clinical & Simple Things

Printed in Great Britain
by Amazon

75408160R00020